Unbound

Raw and Real Plans to Kick Anxiety from Your Bucket List

By

Amanda Plevell, PhD

Copyright 2019 Amanda Plevell
All Rights Reserved.
ISBN: 9781796246803

Everything I do is about bettering our world by making people better. I do that by listening, and then creating things that work. If I listening first, I'm in tune to the reality people believe in, and then I help them learn from it, decide if they want to stay there, or create something new. It is all for growth. If I'm listening now, then it seems noteworthy to have a bit of a discussion about anxiety, a state of the union, if you will. This book has literally written itself through the many, many people I would talk to, randomly meet, run into on vacations, converse with on planes, or swap stories while pushing swings. Everyone has their story. In 14 years in the natural health field, I find it incredible the increase in the number of clients that are coming with anxiety being the number one factor for bringing them in. We are all at some time or another walking around zombie like caught up in the effects of our stories.

It has been estimated that anxiety is now the most common mental illness in the world, even though only about 36% receive treatment, possibly to avoid the stigma associated with "mental illness" or any number of reasons. Also, symptoms vary from an overall feeling of always needing to "do something", to jitters and heart palpitations, to not being able to participate in public, to many many more. The most harmful statistic I read was that even though many are taking medication, they still feel symptoms! But I believe EVERYONE has a right to be healthy and happy, no matter what has occurred in the past. It's not about having a "disease", it's about convincing yourself that you have this same right, and more importantly, that YOU are in charge of it.

It is alarming that so many feel anxiety feelings in our world today, which suggests heavily that we need to look again at our way of living. While certainly nutrition and chemical imbalances play a large part, our conceptualizations hold the largest key to correction. The concepts in this work are based solely on my own experience, both with the experience of anxiety to the point of not wanting to leave the house, as well as my work with clients over the past 12 years. While I will elude to the four forms of anxiety, the majority of this text is based on what I call "Learned Anxiety" and directed specifically to those feeling states of overwhelm and burden to the point where there is such a discomfort they have literally adapted to a sort of "Learned Anxiety", hence the name. In large part this comes down to the intense overwhelm, burden and exhaustion women and men feel, either from their stories of struggle or from carrying the stress of burden of day to day life, or both, all at the expense of their healthy sense of self, and the resultant dis-connect from living, simply because we can't handle one more thing. For the purposes of ease, anytime you see the term 'anxiety' throughout the book, it includes all feelings of over-stress, including overwhelm, burden, helplessness, hopelessness, and the feelings of anxiety associated with them. This is due to the fact that I believe the vast majority of our anxiety comes from a learned helplessness/hopelessness that victimization and/or the perceived sense of who we SHOULD be versus who we sense we ARE imparts. These feelings change the way we view ourselves and the actions we take. Each Limiting Concept we retain keeps us in that place of helplessness and hopelessness, until we are willing to permit an open-ness to consider an alternative.

The goal of this book is not merely to fix things that aren't working. Nothing I say in this book or otherwise should discount the validity of other methods and therapies. In fact, In this book, I will mention four forms of anxiety. While I believe all forms would benefit from what I have learned in working with sufferers, the focus is not intended for clinical anxiety, per se, but more towards what I believe is the most prevalent: Learned Anxiety. I write this book to amplify the focus on embodied solutions that do work. I do not aim to upset the solutions offered by others. Nor should anything I say negate each individual's experience. If we're starting with the wrong questions and limiting beliefs and we don't understand the cause, then even the conventionally right answers will steer us wrong eventually.

When you are focusing on a reality that you don't want you are resisting the totally and completely natural process of letting go and allowing the new. Pain is a natural result of this as is push against that pain. When you are focusing on a reality that you do want that is filled with love and self-awareness and self-respect you shed old layers easily and learn from them, creating better and better along the way as you grow with your experiences. Is the over examination of how things "should" be and the constant push against change that causes a great deal of angst, overwhelm and anxiety. It is this that we are discussing in this book with the intention to drive a greater blessing of being into the world we experience. This is a book for those who want to live a life ripe with experiences of your own choosing.

There is not one RIGHT way, all options are just ONE possible way. As with every source of information, let the seeds of truth take root in your mind that you may transform, and leave those that don't ring true alone. The thoughts I include in this volume, of course, do not replace proper professional attention. In all cases instead of searching for and defining what happened, the question must be asked, "what we can do to bring ourselves to life?

In all forms, I fully believe a new understanding of the concept of" anxiety" is necessary for any who suffer and desire to become "Unbound".

Table of Contents

Introduction : You Are Not Alone 1

Part I: "Its Who I Am"

Raw Truth
You are Not Defective...8

Anxiety is a Protective Mechanism. 9

Anxiety is a Word...9

Real Plan
The Fact, Theory, Fantasy Exercise 11

Part II: "There's Something Wrong with Me"

Raw Truth
Anxiety is a tool 15

Real Truth
Awareness of Your Personal Feelings 16

Part III: "It's a Disease and It's Just How I Am"

Raw Truth
The Feeling of Anxiety 18

Anxiety is a Feeling..18

The Anxiety Monster...19

Judging the Emotion of Anxiety 20

Real Plan
By The End of This Day Exercise

Part IV: " I Don't Know Why I Feel This Way"

Raw Truth
Anxiety is Not Vague 22

Real Plan
Trigger List Exercise 24

PART V: "I Am Not Enough"

Raw Truth
Anxiety and Self Worth
Anxiety is a Disease of Irrationality
Anxiety and Fear 27

Real Plan
Feeling the Wave Situational Technique: 28

PART VI: It's Always Going to Be This Way"

Raw Truth
Anxiety Misuses Creation 29

Fighting Against Anxiety Doesn't Work 30

How Anxiety Heals Us 30

Real Plan
The "I Would Feel Better If" Exercise 32

PART VII: "It's Chemical; It's Genetic; There's Nothing I Can Do"

The 4 Forms of Anxiety 39

Trauma Anxiety 39

Biological Anxiety 43

Situational Anxiety 44

Learned Anxiety 45

Overwhelm and Burden 46

Real Plan
Your Personal Avatar 47

Expectations Worksheet 54

Raw Truth
LET'S GET TO LIVING 56

THE PROCESS IS THE GOAL 56

Using Suggestions of Hope 57
Anxiety is a Law of our Being.. 57
Anxiety and the Wrong use of Force 58
The Importance of Breath and Breathing 58

Real Plan
In the Moment Technique: 59
Anxiety is not WHO you are 59
Emulation Exercise 61
Why Play is important 62
Claiming the Naming 63
Claiming the Naming Exercise 63
Satisfaction's Healing Properties 64
The Difference Between "Gratitude" and "Satisfaction" 64
Happy Action Exercise 67
Gratitude Journal Exercise 68

PART IX: "Other People Don't Struggle Like I Do"

Raw Truth
Anxiety is a Disease of Separation 70
Acts of Service 72
The Comfort Box 74
The No Fear Exercise: 77
Curing Anxiety 79

Real Plan
My List 81
Zen Techniques 84
About the Author 87

1 You Are Not Alone

"She wished he would be quiet and listen to the wilderness within him. Then he might see."

— **Kya, "Where the Crawdads Sing"**

Why do you live where you live? No, seriously, answer the question. Then ask it again. Usually we give ourselves the first prepared answer our minds have in store but when asking it again, we have to give it a little thought before we answer. Ask it again, three, four, even five times. Once we've run through our pat answers, we get down to the heart of the things we usually don't want to admit.

You can do this trick for every deep and meaningful question to find out the true desires of your heart. How often it is that we live our lives believing we are making choices this whole time when much of the time, we are just living off of our pat answers. Do you really want to live where you live? Or is it just where you've always lived? Do you really want to drive what you drive? Or was it the best available option? We HAVE to understand we are creating our life, no matter how it looks like things are stacked against us. And when we look around at our circumstances and environment, it can be hard remembering how we got there, especially when we had such a DIFFERENT plan for our life, or maybe thought it wasn't going to be like this.

When we don't know the answers to these very relevant questions, how do we expect to handle the stressors in life if we aren't even living according to our best self -the very things that nudge up against us telling us we feel so off track from where we

Unbound

thought we'd be?

It's time to get raw and real about what you want in life; to put yourself back in the driver's seat, to kick anxiety and everything else from your bucket list, so you can leave room for getting back to all the things that truly make you happy. Why ELSE do you think you feel the way you feel? You don't do enough of the things that make you sparkle and spend too much time doing the things you think you SHOULD.

Now there are some very real reasons for feelings of anxiety in our lives, but the mechanism of anxiety was meant to be temporary, not the way you live your life!

Let me guess: Everything you've tried so far isn't working right? Still have mood swings, feel up and down happy one minute, sad the next? Do you feel unhappy, or overburdened, exhausted, or overwhelmed? Maybe even completely lethargic, no joy, crying, stressed, anxious and you don't know about what? Do you wake up already burdened with the stress of the day weighing on you? I know how you feel: overwhelmed and overburdened, exhausted at just the THOUGHT of all you have to do today, am I right?

Remember when we were younger and we had all these plans for our adult lives? Success and being somebody, making money, having our own home, the trips we would take, the places in the world we would go, the adventures we would have. Remember feeling wild and free with nothing but time on our sides and the decisions to do whatever we wanted to do that day? Still haven't gotten there? Or maybe you have but you still don't feel the elation and carefree feeling you thought you would have?

Where in life did it change from the wild feeling of this joyful sense of spirit to the drudgery or day to day and tasks? When did anxiety and overwhelm replace the adventures on our bucket lists anyway? I know you've been looking for a doorway that leads to the answers or you wouldn't have picked up this book.

If you've thrown your bucket list out the window, pinned it up on your "someday" board, or have a pinterest board full of vacay locales you never actually intend on going to and titled, "If only", you're in the right place. You probably didn't even realize you added anxiety to your bucket list, did you? And yet it's there. Typical bucket lists mention all the things we want to do before we die. I want to help you create a bucket list in which you learn to LIVE.

We don't even know how we got this way, but suddenly all we feel is stress, the hurried feeling of anxiety, breathlessness and possibly even panic attacks. The first response is to think something is wrong with us and we want to "make it go away". We know we just don't like feeling this way, but we don't know where to start. We first rely physically, on external things that promise to turn our lives around, like supplements, hormone therapies, and drugs.

These may have worked for a while, but guess what, they weren't long lasting were they? Or they caused new problems?

This is why I love what I do so much. Not only does it force me to look at how I want to live, but I get to help other people do the same every day. Whether it's the clients that work with me one on one, or the online community we've created, or the events where we get to hear story upon story, I love to help people find their Greatness Within and release burdens they've needlessly carried a large part of their lives. It usually starts with a person visiting my office due to physical imbalances that they can't see their way out of. But it never is entirely answered in the physical. See the body is a snowball rolling down the hill, once it gets out of balance, it picks up more debris on the way, and I see these effects in every area of their life: relationships, work, family, creativity and more.

I realized that so much about health and balance in all the dimensions in life come from how one FEELS and relates to their life and the bad news is that more and more people are coming in with intense struggles and diagnoses of anxiety and depression and not knowing what to do about it.

Anxiety has such a pervasive nature that it can now be one of the largest categories of medications prescribed. However, the relief is reported to be ineffectual in many cases. It is so pervasive that healing communities of all kinds are having a hard time deciding exactly what is effective and what can be done, and when relief is not felt, determination wanes. It's as though we need to "interrupt our typical programming" because we can't get through when anxiety is pervasive.

But we cannot blanket diagnose all types of anxiety, much of which is actually a highly pervasive stress, overwhelmed feeling of being over-burdened and over pressured. We're not even realizing the start of these feelings in the first place, our energy spent entirely on "what's wrong" and "make it go away". We dive deep into the mental health question in order to discover what happened, and forget the reasons these feelings were brought about in the first place. The pressures for "more" are evident in every arena. We've converted the idea of having a life we love that we live daily and regularly into a someday "bucket list", forgetting that life happens in the journey, not the once in a while experience. Every day regular life has become driven, and to what we usually don't even know, other than that we can say we constantly feel driven to be and do "more". Simon Sinek in his book, "Start With Why" says this, "Peter Whybrow's book "American Mania: When More Is Not Enough" argues that (the reason we suffer) many of the ills that we suffer from today...is the way that corporate America has developed that has increased our stress to levels so high we're literally making ourselves sick because of it. Americans are suffering ulcers, depression, high blood pressure, anxiety, and cancer at record levels. According to Whybrow, all those promises of more, more, more are actually overloading the reward circuits of our brain. The short-term gains the drive business in America today are actually destroying our health."

We've forgotten ourselves at the core and created "selfie" versions that we project to the world, parts and pieces of ourselves we think the world will accept, becoming only parts and pieces of ourselves in the process. Never measuring up in comparison with a world that encourages judgement easily and quickly in the form of "likes" and shares. It's a constant pressure to do more. And it's contagious.

In my opinion, anxiety is a "communicable dis-ease", highly suggestive and contagious. That the feelings and the resulting vibrational patterns of anxiety permeate our culture, giving a reason to explain why we are feeling the way we are. Now more can jump on board as they recognize the same feelings in themselves. Instead of forming a group with like understanding, however, it increases the presence of anxiety as more people now have a "name" to how they feel. Rather than learning to deal with how they feel, they begin to identify with the suggestion of anxiety as a disease, rather than to identify feelings that are saying we're off track. No matter, where it came from or what the cause, the biggest contributor to the problem is this.... we forget that WE are responsible to make any necessary changes, unknowingly putting "anxiety" in the number one position on our bucket lists.

As I mentioned, anxiety is highly suggestive and through suggestion we have seemingly gotten the message that it is something that is permanently wrong with us, it's chemical, it's out of our capable control, it's not something we can do anything about. Sadly, this creates a belief in medication, as opposed to a belief in the self, as the norm. This does the exact opposite of what anxiety needs, the process of: acknowledgement, acceptance, knowledge, decision, confidence in SELF and SELF's abilities and action in the appropriate direction. Just because it works, doesn't make it right. Permanent correction includes suggestions that are focused on the direction of what an individual wants to achieve in themselves, despite the upsets. We have to be cautious with the words we are using so that we're not adding unnecessary "suggestions" to the mix. As helpers to individuals, we need to remind them they are capable and give them the idea they are GOOD at coming up with solutions and support them as they do so. Doing this will help the individual keep clear about feelings, increasing the chances to deal with them effectively and restore a sense of confidence in the ability to be responsible for their life. We need to give new suggestive therapy that leads to a sense of hope. What I'm offering here are new suggestions.

We DO need help to learn how to use anxiety effectively. We don't need to "deal with" anxiety (negotiate, make a deal with) any more than we can "deal with" the electricity that powers our house. Can you tell the outlet to "be nice" and not shock you if you stick your finger in it? NO. You CAN shut the breaker off (the fix, the medicine) but does that mean the electricity stops coming to the house. Anxiety is not a problem. Our chosen use of it is.

In a world where we have the capability to be more connected than ever, we are actually more dis-associated than ever before. I believe anxiety a dis-ease of separation that can be balanced through finding one's place of connection. In my years of practicing in the natural health field, I believe the general feelings of wellness, health, happiness, joy and contentedness extend from a feeling of completion in the self, a wholeness in who one is, and the feeling of being connected to life itself with and for a purpose. Lacking this sense, the cracks between create a sense of separation, damaging the general belief in one's self worth, shaking the core of truth, and leaving room for fears to take root.

Guiding an individual back through the process to connection heavily involves individual understanding, and self-growth, sometimes done alone, and sometimes benefitted with the help of a therapist or person of trust. In any situation where an individual seeks help from a coach, guide, or professional, there has to be a trust, a composite, so it's important that people that work with others can form that connection. They form a composite which forms a trust, and care can continue. This is not only for practitioners, but for the many mothers, fathers, teachers, and people that deal with anxiety with others that could benefit from this work also. I will share my discoveries over the years and why I believe differently about healing it.

We will also learn the forms of anxiety, both, those that are inaccurately believed to make up the majority of anxiety sufferers: Trauma Anxiety, and Biological Anxiety; as well as the most common two: Situational Anxiety, which is dealt with in the moment; and Learned Anxiety, which has feelings of vague-ness and spreads over an extended period of time.

In my opinion, there is nothing currently that has its hand on the throat of our well-being more than the expression of anxiety, stress, and overwhelm, and nothing more capable of developing our growth than learning from it. The number of individuals walking through my door with un-managed stress, anxiety, and/or it's close relative: depression is staggering. Even 10 years ago, it wasn't as common as what we see now.

Why we need to address it is:

- The number of individuals suffering
- The mistaken beliefs about it

- The ineffectual plans for it
- The fact that we can't get anywhere in any other dimension of health or wellness when anxiety is persistent.

*And finally, the fact that I believe that misunderstood anxiety has the potential to progress towards depression, much caused by being unable to resolve the stress causing anxiety. To be sure, anxiety is like the warning light on the dashboard, giving you a chance to fix it. If people are using the word anxiety now, it's the warning light to correct it. Depression is a much more confused state of being, with different chemistry. Depression is much more opaque, more progressed, and keeps us from being the high vibratory evolving beings we are meant to be. It is absolutely imperative we get back to a place of living where stress and overwhelm can be reduced to a point where this slippery slope never begins. In a time where multi-tasking has been held as an asset, it's time to re-prioritize mindfulness and a healthy sense of self.

There IS hope for you. I understand. I've been told I have some unique views on anxiety and because they are not mainstream, and also because of their success in working individually with clients, I'm going to share what RealTime has taught me. It's time to get raw and real about the anxiety you feel so you can create a life experience ripe with adventures of your own making.

You are Not Defective

While it has never been outrightly spoken, society and the use of medicine and the ease of its availability have seemed to be sending us the message that anxiety is bad, undesirable, something to get rid of, rather than understanding the nature of its presence. As if there is something wrong. There IS something that is currently wrong, or feels currently wrong, but it is not YOU that is wrong. YOU are not defective. The situation is. You don't have a DISEASE. You have an improper use of a tool. To really blow your mind, I will tell you that the body, however, doesn't see it as improper. It sees it as proper and necessary and you have been telling it it's WRONG for doing so. How about we thank the body's efforts and see why it feels threatened? What is the challenge we haven't wanted to face? Remember, it is trying to protect you. This is why "getting rid of anxiety" doesn't work, because it is innate in each of us, like a built-in scanner on a computer it is a safety measure, and a necessary one.

Anxiety is a Protective Mechanism.

Anxiety is a protective mechanism. It is not something you "shouldn't have"; it is there innately. It indicates feelings or sensations of danger to self. Problems arise, however, when this is overused, and when the falseness of dangers become seen as a reality. When you next feel anxiety in a situation, determine if the danger is theory, fact, or fantasy (most people link fantasy with a desirable event but sometimes fantasy is also the negative way we use our imagination.) For example: A theory is what someone THINKS is happening. It doesn't make it real. He is theorizing what it could possibly be while you wait to see if it's true. A fact is happening right now. Yes, RIGHT NOW, I'm feeling scared in this waiting room. A fantasy is what you are doing with your imagination while you are waiting in the waiting room. Most often, our minds run away with us rather than dealing with what's really happening in front of us.

Anxiety is a Word

Let's first go over the concept of "Anxiety", so that we can develop a new understanding of it. A new understanding from what one has previously been taught is important in order to break out of the box you've currently been sitting in with it. Many of the ideas in this book will go against current thinking and that's the point. Some will challenge you, some will anger you, and some will be like a lightbulb going off. Pay attention to the ones that cause you to ruffle, as these are indicators that a deep belief is being challenged. This is your cue to look closely at the concept that upset you and see if it is true and/ or useful in your life. Take the points that are useful for your growth in the moment. The following are what I believe about anxiety, especially in the overwhelmed stress related form of Learned Anxiety. Please take and use what feels like truth to you. Also, understand that I am not a medical doctor and make no claims to heal anxiety, diagnose it, or tell you in any way that you do not need medical attention. Use this information as education for yourself and apply what is useful.

The Fact, Theory, Fantasy Exercise

Let's start with an exercise to help clearly define what's going on in your life right now.

First, brainstorm everything that is just going haywire in your life right now. Don't judge it, just right down everything that is bothering you: all your worries, fears, burdens, excesses, and constant thoughts.

_____

_____

_____

_____

_____

_____

_____

_____

_____

_____

_____

_____

_____

Unbound

Next, divide each issue from the previous page into one of three columns:

1. Fact: This thing is happening right now. It's provable.

2. Theory: It's what I logically believe is happening.

3. Fantasy: It's what my mind is imagining.

FACT	THEORY	FANTASY
_____	_____	_____
_____	_____	_____
_____	_____	_____
_____	_____	_____
_____	_____	_____
_____	_____	_____
_____	_____	_____
_____	_____	_____
_____	_____	_____

Most often, you will find that the columns of Theory and Fantasy often intertwine and can be hard to distinguish, and usually make up the largest columns. These columns engage the imagination and the mind and often the realm of the false. Challenging the concepts in these columns is a good way to begin regaining a sense of balance.

Even the Facts column, while tending to be shorter, can be challenged as to the actual truth and validity and you may find that you end up moving them to the other columns. Those that are left in the Facts column can be handled one at a time, individually, with real plans for solution.

2 Let's Begin

We have to understand that in fact, "anxiety" is merely a term assigned to a given set of symptoms. Having experience with myself, a son, and a multitude of clients that have been concerned with this seemingly uncontrollable set of symptoms, it is my opinion that we aren't hitting the problem where it hurts. Once given a name, people claim it as a disease, rather than understand that the feeling of anxiety is actually a tool, a mechanism that the body uses to alert us that something doesn't feel right. We have been trained to believe that it is because something is malfunctioning and "diseased" rather than to work on the problems that are bringing it about. Just because someone has a perpetuation towards "anxiety" doesn't mean they have a "anxiety disease", rather that the anxiety feelings they feel have been given too much power and allowed to overtake the mind, in turn repeating a vicious cycle of physical symptoms. Now, this does not discount the fact that I do believe people suffer from mental illness, I just believe that the vast majority of anxiety symptoms we feel can be dealt with if we learn to balance properly: our bodies and our minds.

Anxiety is COMMON. That does not mean it is NORMAL. For example, let's use thyroid imbalance as an example. We have come to accept thyroid issues as a normal occurrence because so many suffer. I bet you can name at least three people that are having thyroid trouble. The range of thyroid numbers on a thyroid screening panel expand to fit the wide range of people that fall into those parameters, NOT what is healthy or BALANCED for the thyroid. So there are many cases of thyroid imbalance that could have been balanced BEFORE disease states were present. This is my belief and my opinion. Just because so many people suffer from anxiety, that does not mean in my opinion, that it should be accepted. Also, the forms of anxiety vary and we cannot blanket their treatment into one method. It's important to get to know how it feels individually and use it for the tool it was meant to be.

Anxiety is a tool

Anxiety is a wonderful TOOL. It is a balance indicator from your less aware mind to your aware and conscious mind. The body was made to feel anxiety and for the mind to know it so that we would be alerted when something was amiss. Problems arise when these feelings of anxiety rule our lives rather than being a guide we can use to live our lives. Rather than avoiding the problem, we become intimately aware of it. We invite it into our lives and get to know it. Knowledge is power. I know. This sounds like the scary part. We want to know about anxiety LESS. But if you know how it feels for you in particular, you can do something about it.

AWARENESS OF YOUR PERSONAL FEELINGS

Worksheet Exercise

This is How I PERSONALLY Feel. This is how Anxiety affects me.

When it comes to my physical body, I feel it in my…

_____

_____

It feels like (tightness, heat, chills, tension, etc)

_____

_____

If I were to describe the sensations, they feel like….

_____

_____

_____

Without anxiety, I would be/feel….

_____

_____

_____

My life would look like….

_____

Amanda Plevell

3 Feeling Anxiety

Because all anxieties are not the same, there is a large gaping hole in the understanding of what anxiety truly is and must be addressed in order to be an effective resolution according to feelings and actual physiology.

Anxiety is a Feeling

In truth, "anxiety" is actually a word describing a feeling. Over time, the constant feeling of anxiety turned the word into a diagnosis.

I mentioned the true use of the body to develop physiological effects as protective mechanisms and a tool for the individual to change what's happening, like a dashboard warning light. Because of this, I believe anxiety can dramatically become an overuse, or even a misuse of the tool it was meant to be. Is it possible that an individual does not "have anxiety", but rather has a learned imbalance to the response to feeling?

I believe one would help themselves better if they understood that they are currently "feeling anxious". Even if only as a matter of principle. If the body believes everything, we tell it, it would make sense then, wouldn't it, to acknowledge and honor our bodies by acknowledging that we are currently feeling anxious but to not label ourselves as "having anxiety". To do this, tells the body that if we are diseased, we must then always have anxiety. That we are out of power, out of control, and must continue to exhibit symptoms. There is a difference between recognizing a bodily need, and giving it permission to have control over our lives. Please understand, I believe heavily in the use of suggestive therapy, and this is my opinion based on experience, though one should consider the validity of this for themselves.

I want you to also consider the onset of the feelings surrounding the feeling of anxiety. Let's consider the story of my client, whom we'll call Katie.

Katie and the Anxiety Monster

Katie had the opportunity of a lifetime. One she believed would advance her career, make her better at her job, and grow her soul exponentially. When she put in a request for time off and was denied however, a multitude of feelings were present. Injustice, anger, defense, depression, exhaustion, hopelessness, helplessness, lack of power over her own life. Katie had been thinking about seeking out other opportunities for a long time, but this hit the nail on the head.

We talked about how her boss failed her in all the right ways; ways that made her move towards the next growth step for her. It made her shift out of her comfort box. Comfort boxes are the most dangerous places to live because of their ability to halt personal growth. Moving out of her comfort box meant she would face new challenges, but also new levels of evolution.

We also talked about the anxiety monster she was now feeling every day she went to work, which was comprised of her feelings of lack of support, anger at the decision, and the unjust way her boss went about the decision. All that she was feeling wasn't identified as individual feelings and handled accordingly. Instead, the formed this giant what I call "Anxiety Monster" that we run from and are scared of, seeing it as something outside of ourselves. In reality, an anxiety monster is just an immature feeling. It is a toddler having a temper tantrum, because it is based in emotion. Think of any toddler who doesn't have the skills developed yet to handle the anger he feels when you say "no" to the cookie. An Anxiety Monster HAS to throw a temper tantrum and wreak havoc in your life, because it's the only way it knows to get attention for its uncomfortable feelings. It's the little you, the child inside of you that also wants to react out its feelings, because it hurts and they're hard. Think about any child that's acting out. It's actually when they need love the most. They need comfort and the "ok's" that come from a soothing parent. Which is what you are now to your inner child. Let the anxiety monster sit on your lap and hug it. Give it the soothing it needs to understand that yes, your feelings suck. Yes, that situation was awful. But then know that there is a lesson to be learned. Ask how you can grow from what you just experienced. The anxiety monster will go lie back down.

The feelings of anxiety are an incredible growth tool that will get you and keep you on your soul's path, if you listen to it and be aware of it. It is easier to ignore something and try to "make it go away" but permanent benefit comes with awareness and taking it head on. The longer the ignored triggers of anxiety exist, the harder and more buried they become making it more difficult to see where you went astray.

Judging the Emotion of Anxiety

Why are we fearful of the emotion we feel? We don't say, "I'm in love" and then act in fear of it. Or "I'm happy" and then be fearful. Why do we judge the tool of anxiety by saying "I'm anxious", and then determining it's a bad thing? All emotions and feelings were for us to have a human experience. That does not only bring the good feelings but also the "bad".

Perhaps it is because we don't like HOW it feels, but haven't learned how we want to feel instead, assume we should automatically feel that way, or we don't do the things that allow us to feel good. Perhaps we see our happiness as a distant goal that we can't achieve, rather than to see happiness as a process, not as an end result.

Mindset Technique

When you wake in the morning, ask yourself the question, "By the end of the day, how do I want to feel?" This is an easy goal to keep in mind so that throughout the day you can act in ways that bring about this feeling.

4 Anxiety is NOT a Vague Illness

Let's do a quick exercise. Let's brainstorm a list. What are some things that you think are factors in causing anxiety? Where do you think it's stemming from? Hormones? Stress? Nutrition? Worry over kids? Feeling incomplete? Feeling overwhelmed? Insecurities? Fears? Brain chemistry?

Now, looking over our list, let me ask you how VAGUE is anxiety?

See, here is one area I think differently about anxiety: The concept that it's vague. The definition of anxiety is that it is this vague unknown, we don't know WHAT causes it.

I know that one of the very specifics of the definition of anxiety is that there are no known triggers. It is described as being a vague and unknown fear or intense worry. In my opinion, anxiety is there, and it DOES have triggers. I believe some are conscious and some, however, are those we are not aware of, have pushed aside subconsciously, or don't want to acknowledge because they go against our current belief systems and expectations. We generally do KNOW; just don't want to do what it requires. Alternately, we consciously don't know, which means it lies in the realm of the subconscious. If it's in the subconscious, that's an indicator that it's not at the surface of the brain and we need to use strategies to go deeper. There are many books and articles and exercises all over the place with workouts to get to know the subconscious mind and help identify the limiting beliefs so you can resolve them. Remember that the anxiety feeling is there like warning lights. That means it's time to sit down and identify feelings. Take the time to describe HOW you feel. "I feel mad". "I feel embarrassed." " I feel hopeless". Don't use the word "am". This would insinuate that anger is who you are or that you are the kind of person that is embarrassing or hopeless. These are part and parcel fo the negative self-talk we haven't been aware of but need to be in order to heal.

We've never been allowed, or allowed ourselves to take a look at and question our current thoughts, concepts, beliefs, and ways of living. We don't realize it is ALL subject to selection, question, and choice.

When you feel anxiety, the common question is, "Well, to what?" That's just it. If we knew, we wouldn't be feeling it. Whether we know it or not, there are triggers, but identifying them means being willing to look at those triggers. Sometimes, they are the very ones we have shut ourselves off from in protection.

While I tend not to focus more on truth and determination to decide where we want to go next than on the representation or expression of anxiety, it's useful in identifying the form of anxiety by taking a look at any known triggers. Let's take a look at the triggers you are consciously aware of.

My Trigger List:

So far, I know/suspect the following as triggers to anxiety:

1. _____

2. _____

3. _____

4. _____

5. _____

6. _____

7. _____

8. _____

9. _____

10. _____

Now for each trigger, ask yourself where the concept came from. Was there an event or a situation? For example: public places as a trigger.

Concept came from: When I was 5 I had to perform in front of a crowd at school.

Go back to your list and for each, identify if there was a

source. Where did it come from?

1. _____

2. _____

3. _____

4. _____

5. _____

6. _____

7. _____

8. _____

9. _____

10. _____

Now, for each ask yourself what that situation represents, or what was the worst outcome it could be. For example, using the public places example: I was worried I would stutter and everyone would laugh at me.

1. _____

2. _____

3. _____

4. _____

5. _____

6. _____

7. _____

8. _____

9. _____

10. _____

Now, there can be only two realities. That fear you expressed either is truth or it is not. Go through and ask yourself if what you learned is true.

Cross it off if it's false. Next time you feel anxiety and recognize it as a fear from this false list, take a deep breath and say "false". If you do it often enough, you will begin to remember that those concepts are not real.

If you answered "true", then write a new script, make a new plan. What would you do if that did in fact happen? What WOULD you do if they laughed at you? You may find, as you are making a plan, that you see that the fear really is in fact, unrealistic, and you decide to add it to your "false" list.

5 Anxiety and Fear

Anxiety is a close relative of fear. When it comes down to it, if you look at every reason, worry, excuse, or avoidance, it all comes back to fear. There is a fear behind not doing something. Anxiety is based in worry and feelings of something being not quite right, or missing. If you didn't have fear, there wouldn't be anything missing, not measuring up, or amiss.

Discovering what the fear is can be the hard part. I say "can be" because sometimes we hide it from ourselves or don't want to admit to it. You know in your gut what the fear is, but it's difficult to bring it out into the light and see that maybe that truly is a culprit.

The question you can ask to help yourself when you feel anxiety is, "What is the worst thing I fear is going to happen?"

Ask yourself, "Is this a real threat, and a danger to my body that I need to pay attention to?

For example, after my son had a traumatic incident that included an ambulance ride, anytime he would have hunger pains (which to him felt like the same passing out feeling he had) anxiety would crop up in a Situational Anxiety type. He would start hyperventilating, have rapid heartbeat and move to a panic attack. His body was remembering the feeling and responding to the memory of fear. Without being in the same situation, the constructs of his mind made it out to be. I would ask him to ask himself, "Is this a real threat? Am I really in danger?" To this, it would clue him to examine his body and see if there was a real emergency. When he saw it wasn't he could work through the process of bringing himself back down.

The Label, Anxiety, is a Disease of Irrationality.

Threats are felt, as they normally should, but with the feeling of anxiety, remember the snowball effect: threats are perceived everywhere, and then taken to epic proportions. It is NEVER a good idea to attempt to take a person in the situation and tell them what they're feeling isn't true, and it certainly isn't a good idea to do that to yourself. Truth is different to each person, and it certainly FEELS true in the moment. All feelings want to be expressed and paying attention to them is a big step in figuring out the lesson.

The point in understanding that it is a dis-ease of irrationality is to understand that it quickly moves from one thing to multiple things as the imagination moves down the slippery slope with the feeling.

Remember to claim your own imagination. The last question to ask yourself is, "Is this the best use I can put my imagination to?"

ANXIETY REACTS IN THE PRESENT,
BUT WAS BORN IN THE PAST AND FUTURE

Anxiety exists RIGHT NOW, though it is conjuring images of past or future. Even though those time frames don't exist in the present, the feelings of anxiety need to be handled NOW. Fighting against the feeling never works. Instead, let the force move you. Here's an idea

---

Feeling the Wave Situational Technique:

When the feelings of anxiety arise, it's like being in the ocean. Our feet are in the sand and the big wave is coming and our

giddy feelings are high, at least until those anticipatory feelings get overwhelmed and we see the reality of that big wave. Suddenly we panic and turn and run the other way, never getting to experience the joy of the wave crashing sand against our bare feet. Try hold this image in your mind when you feel anxiety but when the feeling starts to feel crushing and overwhelming, allow the crest of the wave to continue on. You'll feel it land at your feet and not knock you down. The success of standing up to the intense emotions will be feelings of strength and get you more and more prepared for handling the overwhelm the next time the wave comes.

Anxiety Misuses Creation

We label "having anxiety" as a bad thing. What many don't understand about people that feel intense anxiety is that they are expressive, ingenious CREATORS. Anxiety is all in the realm of the imagination. We are simply using our creation negatively. Learn how to create your life through imaging and acting as if. Acknowledge your current boundary lines and expand them slowly and progressively. When you have an image, or a goal, of where you want to head in your life, what you want to do, you can begin creating in the direction of your ideal life or situation. These highly creative people especially need outlets where they can create.

Anxiety, remember, is happening in the NOW, but it is being created with past or present in mind. What you think is going to happen is because of past experience or worry about what may come in the future, not about what is currently happening. The feelings are real and present to a situation that doesn't exist. What helps you get through this is the knowledge that anxiety is not a permanent state, unless you claim it. Your tool of anxiety feelings and symptoms may be expressing themselves right now, but you are in charge, and in control of determining if those feelings are indicating a real threat to your being or not. Feel the crest of the wave rise and know that this too shall pass. Fighting the wave doesn't work. The waves EXIST. It's all about how you relate to them.

Fighting Against Anxiety Doesn't Work

Fighting against anxiety is like fighting against yourself, hating your Self, and distancing your Self from that part of your Self. How can you learn to love yourself and be yourself (which is how anxiety heals us) if you hate a part of yourself? Feeling the feelings of anxiety is an acknowledgement that you don't like certain parts and feeling a learned helplessness. It's an opportunity to re-direct your life through different actions than what you've acted on before. Feelings of anxiety are a way to heal that which is wrong.

How Anxiety Heals Us

Did you hear when I said, "How anxiety heals us"? That's because the feelings of anxiety are not there for no reason. They are there to alert us that we are off track, and that something doesn't feel right. I fully believe that anxiety can be felt when our natural lives are not in alignment with our souls. Perhaps we are living up to expectation, or attempting to anyway. Either way, we are not living the way we know in our hearts to feel satisfying.

Pushing anxiety away as if it doesn't exist, or take drugs to "get it to stop" may be a temporary fix, but the key word here is "temporary". Sure, it may help in the beginning, but in my experience, the longer you push something off, the worse the symptoms are. And they may NOT be in the same way that they originally started. This escalation of long-term symptoms morphing into other parts of the life and body makes people believe they are very unhealthy rather than to go back and address the original problem. The solution thus gets farther and farther away and more buried. It is important right away to feel that wave's crest, admit we feel it, and determine that anxiety is a powerful tool that we can use in our favor rather than against us.

Anxiety is not your shadow side, the negative side of you, or your evil twin. It is a protective ally, determined to keep you safe. These protective systems are innate and powerful but like all things, work best in your favor if they are in BALANCE. Using the yin/yang symbol is a good reminder of balance in your life. You can't have the "good" without the "bad", the black without the white, the light without the dark. Most importantly, not only do these opposites exist, they are ever flowing in, out, and around each other. Meaning these energies are not stagnant. All that you feel succumbs to the verbage "this too shall pass". When all the pieces of your life are allowed to work in harmony, there is balance.

We have to address the triggers...which ultimately comes down to the fears. What you BELIEVE is going to happen is usually worse than what IS happening. Again look to assess the truth in the fear. Fears take away your power/control, and ultimately that is what we are anxious about . Usually anxiety happens because we are trying to control how WE want it, trying to defend against any "bad" thing that can happen. Learning to let go, and have faith and trust in the situation are useful exercises for those that struggle. If we're feeling struggle, often times it's because the answers aren't there yet and we need patience for the development.

During this stage, we use a couple exercises with my clients that can help change the direction of your thoughts from the problem to the solution.

The "I Would Feel Better If" Exercise

This exercise is a simple brainstorm answering the question: "I would feel better if…"

Now, are there any things you can do right now, to start bringing some of these about?

The Original "Why" Exercise

In order to get a better understanding of what we're working with this is your one and only chance to prove to me WHY your life is so hard. On the left side of the page, write down all the things you do that occupy the time of your day. On the right side, write down WHY you do that particular thing.

My Doing List	Why I Do It
_____	_____
_____	_____
_____	_____
_____	_____
_____	_____
_____	_____
_____	_____

Amanda Plevell

Once you see in front of you all of the ways you spend your day, it's easy to see the things that are maybe unnecessary for you to do, especially if the particular WHY you do it is out of fear or limiting belief, or a sense of false responsibility, or to "prove" who you are to someone.

The trick then to be more in accordance with who you want to be, living out the life you want to live, is to come up with the real WHY you do anything. Why does it matter to you?

Can't get your family to follow along with your program? CAn't get your kids to do what you're asking, your spouse to share in responsibilities? Your employees to be motivated to perform?

True leaders in companies and organizations know that the reason why they are so successful is because they inspire people with their WHY. They are clear on WHY they do what they do, and their product is simply a projection of that, and the result is an intense clear vibration that attracts people that have been looking to feel that way. . Leaders elicit a loyalty because their people buy into the WHY of what they are doing, not WHAT they are selling.

Simon Sinek speaks to this more fully in his book, "Start With Why", if this is a theory that calls to you and you desire to define your business more clearly and improve your practices. But, in the meantime, I fully believe this principle can be applied in the personal life as well as the professional. Sometimes the reasons we do something can be unclear to someone else. They may not understand why the back of the toilet seat needs to be wiped, or why you vacuum every day, or why towels are folded a certain way. They don't know you are trying to keep sanitation a high priority, or because that's the only way the towels will fit in the drawer. They don't receive the vibration of these loftier and logical goals, they receive the vibration of "not enough-ness" due to your intensity of anger and frustration.

To correct this simple mis-alignment of energy fields, it would be wise for you first to know WHY you do those things you deem important. It might be that you decide they aren't all that important in the first place, and that you are simply following old conditioning, at which point you might decide to update your ideas of what IS truly important.

Second, it is time to get yourSELF into alignment with the real WHY you do anything. Dig deep taking a look at yourself and ask yourself what it is you are trying to accomplish and why. "I love my family so much and I want them to be as healthy as they can be. I am a good steward to our home and I LOVE that people feel at home here. I want people to kick off their shoes and relax, feeling safe and comforted, so we can all together feel relaxed and enjoy fun times together. I picture games played around this table, and all of us sitting around the couch comfortable watching movies, preparing healthy snacks together, laughing and enjoying each others' company. I see us snuggling and reading books, or pulling out the photo albums and reminiscing", sounds MUCH better and FEELS much better vibrationally, than "I have all this work to do and YOU aren't helping and you never help me and you just cause stress in my life by making my life harder! You don't play your part and you are not responsible", doesn't it? Chances are very good that your family has NO IDEA why you do the things you do, and rather than spending your energy trying to make them see and agree with you, perhaps you want to get clear on the activities and the feelings you want to create in each of your spaces. You must have an understanding of your vision clearly, so that your family can picture it with you. But you seeing it clearly will create a different vibration that YOU are projecting and law of attraction can raise others to that same vibration. It could help to engage the family and envision what EACH person is thinking these home spaces are for, because they might have different ideas and could be the cause for why there is discord: there is no agreement, no shared image.

Take a look at each area of your home or property and decide what its use is: what activities will be done there, and how you want the individuals in them to feel. Share your family this image of what you see happening in each space, imagining the activities and how the people feel, and most importantly, WHY this matter to them. It could be "I imagine you and your friends playing games, and sharing food here, having a good time. I imagine us sharing movies in this room (and go into detail of how that feels) Get everybody excited about what this could look like so that they buy into your WHY. That, coupled with the high vibration coming from you, and you could just find that you inspired people without even trying.

So now, take a minute to do just that. Use the next page to get a firm clarity of your WHY, whether it be in your home or anywhere else. This is available on the UnBound website also, so that you can do this multiple time as needed.

Your New WHY Exercise

Unbound

6 The 4 Forms of Anxiety

So far, we have been working in the conscious realm, the things we can think through. Now I said earlier that often the feeling of anxiety is not in the conscious mind, which is why there is the feeling of "vague-ness". This teaches us a "learned anxiety". This is often where the majority of the work needs to be,

However, we first we have to rule out PTSD because if there is a known traumatic pin-pointable situation, we need to address the trauma, and then address the subconscious limiting beliefs that were created with that trauma. Which brings us to the first of our forms of anxiety: Trauma Anxiety.

Trauma Anxiety

Most trauma anxiety comes from a definite and definable incident or occurrence. The resulting behaviors stem from the fear that the trauma will happen again, or the limiting concepts that the trauma taught them.

An interesting occurrence I've come to understand in working with individuals is that we all have our traumas, some are just more extreme than others but that does not rule out their level of affect. One trauma that we would call extreme can have little to no effect on another. Some traumas that seem minor can have just as hard an impact as one that is known to be major. It's like that quote you have no idea someone else's struggle, so be kind. And don't minimize other peoples' traumas. You don't get to decide how someone should feel. What they feel is what is true for them, no matter how irrational it sounds to you. Think about the child who believes there is in fact a monster under his bed. We KNOW this is not true. HE does not. It is, in fact, very very real to him. Seeing the fictional monster had to have been very traumatic in his mind, just as yours are to you. The key in any trauma is to not let our response to trauma be more traumatic than the trauma itself. We also have to be open to understand the possibility that for every perceived threat or injury that person or situation failed you in exactly the ways they needed to fail you. Your own growth will be determined by your openness to the ability to take "victim" out of your mindset.

We also have to use caution in trauma type anxiety, because the point is not to come up with new diagnoses, or places to "blame" the feeling. Again, "suggestion" is highly powerful and we do not want to give more bondage to an already difficult situation. For example, I worked with a girl who was in counseling due to family trauma she suffered. The words she heard constantly concerned how she was a "trauma child" and how we needed to work with her. These are the suggestions she received constantly from her trust sources, which had a heavy impact on her belief in her recovery. However noble are the best intentions through counseling and therapies of different kinds we fail to see how the diagnosis and continued discussion can KEEP an individual in trauma. There is a time to work through the trauma with the intent being on changing the limiting beliefs that would keep one traumatized. We also HAVE to see that though a trauma brain looks different, it DOES NOT have to stay that way, and this is so through new experiences and new understandings. We need to develop new suggestive therapy that gives suggestions that lead to hope.

But Isn't Anxiety and/or Depression due to Chemical Imbalance?

Now is about the point where people ask me "What about Chemistry"? What I believe is different. Yes, I believe trauma of any kind will change the chemistry of the body, but what I believe differently is that it can change AGAIN. It's not a deficiency in the body being able to produce chemicals in balance, it's because the body has a defense mechanism, chemicals are produced for protection.... but then they get stuck there! Either by avoidance, distractions or drugs, or not addressing them, identifying the situation and dealing with it. See the body made feelings of anxiety as an adaptation. We made it a disease. As long as we treat it as a disease (biological or genetic) it won't be cured. Once we start seeing it as a dis-ease, an awareness and a separateness from the truth within you, we can heal it.

See, we've created it as a THING. Now is where I will warn you as I did in the beginning about potential concepts that could be upsetting. Here is a section where people tend to feel a little ruffled. It's almost like, once defined, people want to keep their diagnoses and hold them as something that finally made sense for them. It gave them a reason. An understanding. Now this is not true for everyone, but I wonder how often people then live their lives according to this definition they've accepted for themselves. My worry, as a warrior, myself, is that I believe diagnoses originally to be used to define what's wrong IN ORDER TO CORRECT IT. There is a great danger in using it as a definition of who one IS and staying there. It also runs the risk of being an excuse to not be the best one can possibly be. I challenge all to not let anything be something that stands in your way of your own Greatness Within. I tell you what, we've got to teach people their specialness, their Greatness Within in other ways.

Understand this, the word is really a feeling, but we've made it into an existence. It does NOT mean it's in your head, and that what you've been through isn't warranted. But I don't believe in taking away any person's power to heal and change it into something new. It is NOT set in stone. Situations may make it HARDER, but it is unfair of us to put people in boxes where they believe a better life in IMPOSSIBLE.

With all of this discussion and attention on this manifestation we've created, my worry is this: That kids now toss the word around and understand it as a "thing they have" even though they don't really understand it. They know it to be a disease that needs medication. "I have anxiety" We have to change that. "It's possible you are feeling anxious. Let's look into that" We've put attention on it, we've given it a name whereas before it was just a feeling, and then we haven't well taught people to deal with the feelings. We teach them to cover them up. How have you covered it up? Sometimes how you've covered it up can give clues as to the underlying problem.

Sometimes, our anxiety stems from an occurrence that was traumatic or otherwise stressful at the time but we never learned to grow through it. Much of our held anxiety is from situations and feelings we haven't learned to let go of yet. Our goal in coaching or counseling through Trauma type anxiety should be to learning peace over what happened. While learning skills for "coping", we will still need to develop for skills to learn peace. Not because the other person that hurt us should be absolved of responsibility but for the known fact that forgiveness and making peace is for the victim, not for the perpetrator anyway. We have to be careful that we are not keeping the trauma alive. There are basically two trains of thought on trauma protocol: To examine and analyze who, how, why, when a situation happened. Or alternately, to decide where we're going to take it and what we're going to do with it. It would seem to matter less to discover the how and why than to learn the path to moving forward. In my opinion, when we are trying to analyze the hows and whys of why someone would do something, we're really just looking for warranted evidence that agrees with our sense of self: that we are less than, not worthy, or somehow deserving of pain. We are each individually none of these things. Anxiety, I believe, can stem from one of two things: self-worth, and fear.

Timber Hawkeye was a practicing monk and said it this way.

"The event that initially angered us happened in the past, and the person who upset us is possibly no longer in our lives. Bus as long as we continue mulling over past experiences, essentially re-living them in our minds and bodies, we will keep experiencing them over and over again and never fully recover. By believing, re-living, and repeating the elaborate story that we constructed around the initial feeling, we keep the emotion alive, and it burns inside of us for years to come. It feels very real to us, but it's only a memory of a feeling felt long ago. It's best to think of the memory of our pain as a scar, which will remind us of where we've been without dictating where we're going."

Biological Anxiety

Next, and alongside physical chemistry, we address any other potential physical factors. There's also a form of anxiety we look for when I do appointments at my office and that is Biological Anxiety, where a food or irritant (bacteria, pathogen, virus, toxin) is causing a feeling of stress in the body. I've seen kids with responses to red dye, gluten, wheat, sugar, additives, and more. What happens physically in the body has a direct effect on all expressions of the body, including how one feels.

I completely believe that every endeavor towards health needs to start in the gut. The gut is 80% responsible for your immune system, is completely responsible for your food digestion (which are the nutrients that feed every part of your body and brain), and 60% responsible for your immune system (which defends your body against invaders, some of these being food and the bacteria that came in on your food). Every part of the body that needs to produce something else for the body relies on a healthy gut to do this. For example, the gut is 95% responsible, according to Fit Life TV, for serotonin production. If you want to be happy, get healthy! And it all starts in the gut!

I've always said, health doesn't have to be hard. If the body's cells are receiving nutrients, and the body can eliminate waste from the cells on out, there is no reason for inflammation, and inflammation is the root of all symptom and all disease. Just make sure you are taking in nutrients to the best of your ability, and encourage your body's elimination. Let the body work itself back into balance before you take drastic measures, assuming it, itself, is the problem. Make sure to balance two areas of your Self: give your body's basic functioning some assistance (as opposed to interference) and deal with your concepts that could be keeping you in your current state. There are basic and simple physical things you can do to help your body align itself. Between taking care of the body, and dealing with your concepts, you will find how to balance the tool of anxiety and get on with creating your life rather than letting it bounce you back and forth.

There is a form of chemical anxiety felt physically in the body due to stress of withdrawal from a substance like drugs, alcohol, even foods. I don't separate it as its own category due to the fact that there was a reason for the addiction to begin in the first place and it's necessary to get back to ground zero in order to look at the origination of Trauma or Learned Anxiety.

Situational Anxiety and Learned Anxiety

Having acknowledged direct trauma or physical factors, to be most useful we can next address whether the response is Situational or Learned Anxiety.

Situational Anxiety

Situational Anxiety is what the body sees as acute trauma or stress. It's happening right now. This is where management techniques can be used. Situational Anxiety can be a re-occurrence of a past trigger or it can be an entirely new situation in someone that isn't prone to feelings of anxiety, but the new situation warrants it. So that the new situation doesn't become a "trauma", we have to effectively reflect back and deal with our feelings of the event. A "re-triggering" of a previous event indicates that there is more to understand about that previous stressful situation.

In the Moment Technique:

In the moment of an anxious situation, try chewing gum. The act of chewing makes the body focus on the act of digestion. Chewing gum is a psychological trick that tricks the mind into thinking it is safe. "If I'm eating, I must be safe", the brain says.

*Be cautious however not to use food for this.

*Using this technique is useful in the moment, but still needs the long-term restoration of working through the feelings of anxiety.

Learned Anxiety

Learned anxiety is the chronic vague feeling, just knowing something isn't right, constantly. It's still situational, it's just that unmanaged situational has added up to a chronic vague feeling, so you still break it down into the multi-situational issues. Learned anxiety is an indicator to get to know oneself better and find out where your life is differing. Here is yet another area in which my approach to anxiety differs: I believe anxiety always comes down to: Living one way, while desiring to live another way. It is essential to look at what you wanted life to be, and what you currently are living. Harmony between who you are and the kind of person you want to be is absolutely essential. If you make choices that sound "logical", then the mind can rationalize your actions, however, your heart won't understand and then you are living divided, fighting a war inside yourself, which is the most difficult kind of war to wage.

While there are those that associate "Anxiety" with trauma as the main culprit, I believe the most prevalent form of anxiety we have is Learned Anxiety. Learned Anxiety can step from any of the other 3 types of anxiety in that the individual figures out, however ineffectively, to keep moving on, though not in the peaceful sense of letting go, but in an unhealthy forceful determination.

Overwhelm and Burden

The most common source of Learned Anxiety, is the anxiety of stress, overwhelm, and burden. In my experience this is the most common, most pervasive, most prevalent, and most relevant to the situation of those that might be reading this book. Overwhelm, the feelings of pressure, demands, expectations of life and reality can develop a long-term stressful pattern that can be just as damaging as the protective mechanisms developed through Traumatic Anxiety.

It is largely related to all our own concepts, our thoughts and beliefs. The key is to know ourselves well, our core values, and make decisions according to them. Then we need to approve of our own decisions instead of waiting for signs of approval from others.

People feeling anxiety pigeon hole themselves into ALL the ways they don't measure up and their perceived failures, rather than seeing one incident as a challenge. All of us struggle and we need to see the incidences as singular, not personal, and not as evidence of our failures.

As you move through the waves cresting at your feet, you will learn they do in fact fall at your feet and don't wash over you and out of existence. These tools are all so that you can live your life with greater ease. Allow yourself to read the thoughts in this book again and again so that you can start changing your view, and thus the way you speak, about what anxiety is. Determine to take control of what it is you want for your life. It is absolutely imperative to get in touch once again with the various roles you are choosing to play in your life. This is handled by determining your perception of expectations: of yourself, others, and what they might in turn expect out of you. Then it is necessary to determine true responsibility for the various activities you may have claimed as your own. But first, addressing feelings of anxiety is much more effective if you are coming from a place of confidence in knowing thyself. Remember, anxiety is often bred from fear and low self worth. It is necessary to determine your core values and who you want to be as a person. We call this exercise "Capturing Your Personal Avatar" because you are used to playing to an illusion. It is easier if you create a "character" of who you see yourself as and who you want to be, so that you can "watch" your life play out in front of you, being more objective and taking situations less personally. Practicing your avatar allows you to play the role you are choosing, while essentially "growing into the role". It is the single most important exercise to do to regain a sense of confidence and clarity over your life, creating a life that is ripe with adventures of your own making.

Your Personal Avatar Exercise

Write down who you are, who you want to be. You get to decide this! What are your core values? What is the kind of person you want to be? How do you want to feel? How do you want people to see you? What effect do you want to have on the world? Harmony between who we are and the kind of person we want to be are essential to our sense of peace. Only then will we not experience a sense of anxiety, because our actions will be in alignment with our values. It might really help you to do this exercise which is available on our website: https://drfoodie.live/blogs/wellbeing/capturing-your-personal-avatar

To be successful with ANY role in ANY area of your life, the most important factor is that you have a good grasp on WHO you are and that you DON'T FORGET IT!

This sounds easy enough but can be an overlooked step, especially if you are one who tends to give of themselves until their own teacup is empty, forgetting to refill it along the way. This is especially for those who tend to give their all to everyone else.

Keep in mind there is a BIG difference in selfishness vs self-respect. Selfishness is putting your WANTS before someone's NEEDS. Self-Respect is putting your own NEEDS before someone else's wants.

As caregivers, as caring loving compassionate people it's easy to forget this and end up a puddle on the floor, overwhelmed and overburdened, and completely bound up. You might definitely want to check into the UnBound book and conference for more help with this!

To feel like you are living the person you want to be in each role of your life it's important to know who that person is. Then, you live, breathe, move, talk, and act from that image. Which is why we do this exercise called your "Personal Avatar". It's the image of who you see yourself to be.

If you are constantly only giving to the needs and wants of others, what you have to offer the world can very quickly be misconstrued and forgotten because all of your time, effort, and energy is taken up, leaving no time to fulfill your greatest purposes. If you represent yourself inaccurately in order to take care of others' WANTS, sooner or later that very person with whom you have created the desired relationship will discover that you misrepresented yourself, and one or both of you end up feeling bad.

The best thing you can do is honor yourself for who you really are. This is what will show true to others and ultimately bring you the happiness you are looking for.

If you are newly out of a relationship, or a transition, or a new job, this is an important exercise to complete as you discover who you are outside of that role and where you are going from here, so be sure to re-visit this exercise repeatedly throughout your life.

It's time to be very clear with yourself and write an image of yourself, to develop your persona, your character, your Personal Avatar.

An image is the "movie" you are playing of yourself. It is who you see yourself to be and hopefully who you are portraying to the world.

If you want people to be in love and connected with you, you best be in love and connected with yourself. Like we said earlier in the "Original Why" exercise, people get behind you because of the vibration they feel from the authentic living of your WHY, your understanding of who you are and why you do what you do.

The IMAGE:

Use the following prompt questions to help you write a complete image on who you see yourself to be and what is true for you. Write, use words, draw pictures, paste pictures, whatever you need to do to get a good image of who this person is, exactly. Remember to answer these questions according to who you WANT to become (and are already in the process of whether you realize it or not). When you answer these questions, consider your WHY, the thing that drives you, and the kind of person you want to be.

For example: After spending some clarity time with myself and considering the following questions, I can pull together a basic statement to live by, which can change as you evolve, by the way. My WHY: "Everything I do is to help people be the best they can be, to see their Greatness Within and love who they are, see their value and what they have to offer. I act in ways that people to feel valued when they're in my space. I intend that my children are encouraged by me to be successful in themselves, responsible and capable. I decide to feel content and satisfied, purposeful and useful and choose to do things that feel good to my growth."

People can get behind your WHY not because they agree with you even, but because they will feel the powerful vibration of your clarity.

The Questions:

1. This is how I see myself as a person

2. These are the things I like to do

3. If I had an hour to myself this is what I would be doing

4. I want people to think this of me...

5. People say I am...

6. I am proud of...

7. These are the things I am good at.....

8. These are the groups I want to be part of....

9. My friends say I am

10. When I was a child I enjoyed

11. This is how I spend my day

12. The kind of work I do

13. The kind of work I enjoy

14. This is how I see myself looking like.

15. This is how I like to dress...

16. This is what people think of me

17. These are my skills, and talents, and characteristics…

18. I am…

19. I believe….

20. I like to sleep like this, eat like this, act like this...

21. This is what time I like to wake up....Go to bed....

22. These are activities that are absolutely important to me to do....

23. How do I want to feel?

24. How do I want to present myself to my team/colleagues/family?

25. How do I want to be as a mom?

26. How do I want to be as a wife?

27. How do I want to be as a (every role of your life)?

28. These are my core values…

29. This is the kind of person I want to be...

30. Any other details about how you want to see yourself.

One you have created your Personal Avatar, you LIVE, BREATHE, ACT LIKE, TALK LIKE, REPRESENT YOURSELF LIKE how this Personal Avatar would.

What can be the most helpful is that in each moment, look around and assess what role is being required of you. Ask yourself these three questions every time you step into a new role throughout your day:

1. What role am I in THIS moment?
2. How do I want to perform this role? (How do I want to feel, and what do I want others to feel from me?)
3. How does my image (my avatar) respond in this situation? What is the kind of person I want to be and how do I want to represent myself?

Expectations

After deciding who you are choosing to see yourself as, it is time to look at the current expectations and responsibilities you have accepted into your life.

Many times, anxiety is unknowingly coming from expectations and societal pressures from our peers, our families, our communities, our beliefs and religions. For sure, the feelings of overwhelm and overburden would benefit from this exercise as definitely we feel responsible to so many things, beings, and entities that we are muddying our clarity with what we believe others expect of us. It is good to address is on paper so we can see it out in front of us. Many times, the expectations aren't even true, and those people really don't expect that of you. Also, when we see them laid out, we can see how big they look and make decisions about which are those we want to feel responsible for and which we don't. Often, we act according to these expectations rather than what we know to be true for US. I would challenge everyone to utilize the Expectations Activity below just as a way of "tidying up" your role in each person's life. Those in anxiety of overwhelm and burden tend to way overtake on things that aren't their responsibility. We get anxious and irritated believing it's the other person, when really it's our own inability to say no from a place of truth within ourselves and has nothing to do with the person "irritating" us but the fact that we are susceptible to irritation.

If you feel like your cup is empty from pouring it out to others all the time maybe you're filling it from the wrong kettle. Hear this: when you are living, acting, and breathing from your Greatness Within, that place that is at one with God Source Life Love, that kettle is constantly filling your cup so much to overflowing. It's that overflow that seeps out to others, all on it's own. It's that extra happiness that boils over into your relations with others. It's the satisfaction and content that oozes into every cell of your body. It's the overflow that makes you be able to give of yourself consistently without feeling depleted. Fill up your cup with the kettle of source and you'll never run dry.

When you feel anxiety that could be expectation related, ask yourself what is it you WANT to be doing right now, despite societal expectations? Then ask yourself why you are following the path of expectation, and what you hope to gain from it. You can also find this Expectations Activity on drfoodie.live as well as the Reverse Expectations Activity, which allows you to analyze what expectations YOU have of OTHERS. Finally, access on the same site the Expectant Self Activity, which allows you to analyze what YOU expect of YOU.

Unbound

Expectations Worksheet

On the left side of the following worksheet, write a list of all of the people that you feel have expectations of you, including yourself. On the right side, write down what those expectations are. See the example below. Do this for every person that has an impact on your life.

Person #1   **Expectation**

17-year-old son   Cook his meals

                             Wash his clothes

                             Makes his costumes for school

                             Proofread his homework

Person 2   **Expectations**

4-year-old daughter   cook her meals

                             Wash her clothes

                             Be at her beck and call

Now, go through the list of expectations and cross off any expectations that you don't choose. You can recognize which ones are truly YOUR responsibility, and which ones aren't. If you feel they ARE your responsibility, ask yourself why someone else's things are your responsibility. If you are having trouble deciding WHO should be responsible for WHAT, I highly recommend that you access the lesson entitled Responsibility on DrFoodie.live.

You can also see that the expectations are and should be different for the different aged people in your family. Some is appropriate and sometimes it is necessary to move the responsible party into his own responsibility. A good formula for this is:

Capability + Skills = Responsibility.

Is the person capable (physically, mentally, emotionally) and do they have the skills? If so, they can be responsible for the task. It is one thing to do something for someone out of kindness and to make their lives easier, but not at the expense of your own wellbeing (or theirs).

Is your preschooler able to get his own breakfast? If he had the skills, could he? Could you set bowls, spoons and cereal boxes in his reach so he could be successful on his own? Do you always want to be washing his hands for him or do you want to teach him how to do it? Set up the environment for his success. You will thank yourself when you see the pride, he has in being able to do things for himself.

Don't let your self-talk get to you about "you should", etc. Just be honest with yourself and in comparison, with the image you have for yourself circle the expectations you can agree to and want to do, and cross off the ones you don't. There is no such thing as "have to". There are plenty of people you can make arrangements with if you truly hate doing laundry.

The circled ones are your new image with that person. Stand firm and be willing to say no when they expect something from you that is not what you want for yourself. Transition them by saying, "This is your responsibility and I have faith in you."

7 WHAT YOU CAN DO: LET'S GET TO LIVING

You will notice in working with me that while there is a time for everything, I am not heavily invested in spending time on the "what was" or even "what is" other than to use both experiences as direction. This is also why I don't discuss Trauma Anxiety in detail in this book. Many times, people need to experience the level of pain and spend time there until they are ready to release the victim. This is one time where counseling professionals are the highly equipped people that may be just what the individual needs for the time being.

If I take my clients through a memory, there is a specific purpose for it, but most often, we get to the business of living and let the past creep up for healing as it comes up during the process.

THE PROCESS IS THE GOAL

First of all, understand, the PROCESS is the GOAL, not the end result of "not having anxiety". You will always have the tool. But you will learn how to use it. Anxiety means you have the opportunity to get strong, allow change and transformation. It is the learning process that is of value. The allowing, the willingness to change, to see a new idea, and transform your life due to this willingness that is what we strive for. This is where the learning happens.

To begin restoring your balance, it is essential to gain some new understandings about the use of the term.

Using Suggestions of Hope

Anxiety is highly suggestive and through suggestion we have seemingly gotten the message that it is something that we can't control, it's chemical, it's out of our capable control, it's not something we can do anything about. This does the exact opposite of what anxiety needs - confidence in SELF and SELF's abilities. We DO need help to learn how to use anxiety effectively. We don't need to "deal with" anxiety (negotiate, make a deal with) any more than we can "deal with" the electricity that powers our house. Can you tell the outlet to "be nice" and not shock you if you stick your finger in it? NO. You CAN shut the breaker off (the fix, the medicine) but does that mean the electricity stops coming to the house. Anxiety is not a problem. Our chosen use of it is.

Anxiety is a Law of our Being.

Anxiety is a defense mechanism, a tool for use by the body and mind. It is innate in us, meaning we didn't have to do anything to instill ourselves with tools and mechanisms, they are there and we are born with them, just like the baby's natural reflex to turn to breastfeed and suck without being taught.

Because this is innate, and omniscient and ever present, trying to break this law doesn't work. This anxiety mechanism is a principle of our existence. It then is a LAW of our being. We can't break the universal law. When we try we only break ourselves against the law.

Picture the force of the river. If you try to swim upstream, who gets beat down and exhausted...you or the river? You have two choices: turn around and go with the flow, or get out into a new environment where the conditions are different. Trying to FORCE anything to happen just creates more feelings of anxiety. Go WITH the force instead of opposing what IS.

Anxiety and the Wrong use of Force

Sometimes we can feel anxiety because we are forcing something to happen. This is a good time to take a step back, stop what we are doing, breathe and stop thinking about the situation. Allow chi, or life energy to be felt moving through the body and out into your life. Once you feel more relaxed and moved by the chi, energy, or spirit inside of you, then you can get back to work with the perspective of the spirit. This means to stop trying to direct, control, manipulate or "make something happen". When you are guided into action, it will be the right timing. In the meantime, the breath is a tool that is rooted in the presence. Allowing oneself to return to a state of the present is to allow oneself clarity of mind to direct right action, right now.

The Importance of Breath and the act of Breathing

Ever get upset when someone tells you to "just breathe" to get through anxiety or a panic attack? Author Danny Dreyer in "ChiRunning" offers a clearly stated answer as to what physically happens when we shallow breathe, the type of breathing we use during an anxiety attack. "Shallow breathing activates the sympathetic survival instinct of flight or flight response. This, in turn, stimulates stress receptors and increases your heart rate. The right of flight response triggers the release of the stress hormones cortisol and adrenaline, causing the body to burn blood sugar and store fat. It also raises your blood pressure as a result of the lower oxygenation rate of your muscles, which ultimately overloads the adrenal glands and breaks the body down." Ever feel chronic fatigue, low energy, worry, cardiovascular concerns, heart palpitations? Been told you have adrenal exhaustion, need B vitamins, possible thyroid problems, etc? Perhaps you just received a possible explanation. Breathe! The Unbound website has useful exercises and lessons in breathing.

Many times, anxiety arises and we engage in a vicious cycle of behavior. We seem to think we can "think our way out" which really just causes more turmoil. The key is to STOP, follow the above paragraph to learn to BREATHE and engage for a time in something else. It is wise to choose a meditation or practice. Thinking your way out doesn't work, but focusing the mind does. Stop analyzing and focus the mind in a practice that motivates you, frees you, and works towards bettering yourself, ASIDE from the situation at hand.

In the Moment Technique:

You might try deep breathing techniques, or "Nadi Shodana" which is an alternating breathing technique to awaken and align both hemispheres of the brain. This powerful technique gives your body and hands something to DO, while focusing the mind on an action, all while it brings you back to the present.

With a child, you might consider blowing bubbles, or breathing through a straw which will focus and direct their breathing through the tighter air passage of the straw, which takes focus. You can have them blow a cotton ball across a table, or blow ripples into a bowl of water.

Anxiety is not WHO you are

As we've already discussed, there is a difference between "anxiety" and "feeling anxiety". Anxiety is not who you are and neither is "feeling anxiety". Anxiety doesn't need to be a description of who you decide yourself to be. Because everyone has this protective mechanism built in, does everyone "have anxiety" then? It is all in how you choose to use it. We decide how to feel in any moment, not the situation or what's happening around us. Perceiving that there is a "way" we "should" be acting through a moment is playing to the crowd, not from the truth within. Feelings are normal and happen in the moment. We learn from them. Emotions contain a memory of a feeling . These are often the things that can lie to us as we exaggerate or dramatize the memory. For example, If you were to discuss with someone a very hard situation that they experienced, if you witness you can visually see their shoulders droop and feelings come over their face. It is as if they are living the situation again. It is as if they are going through the feelings, even though it is not happening RIGHT NOW. They are feeling emotion: the memory of a feeling.

Feelings of anxiety are only a PIECE of your emotional makeup. It is not WHO you are.

Each person responds differently to different situations and how it feels to them. But you do get to decide HOW you want to let the situation make you feel. You do get to decide what you will take from the situation. We ALL are going to have experiences that are lesser, and some that are more enjoyable. People handle them differently. But if you haven't liked how you've been handling those that come into your life, try observing people that you think handle it better. Each person has their own struggles, but they may have grown in an area you can learn from, again not as a comparison to how "wrong" you are doing it, but in an effort towards growth.

Amanda Plevell

Emulation Exercise

A good exercise here would be to grab a pen and paper and write down the people you admire and/or emulate. Write down why you admire them.

Who: _____

What I admire about them:

_____

_____

_____

_____

_____

_____

_____

It's important to see what you write, because typically these are the things you think you DON'T have. Additionally, we've already discussed how important it is to create a new confident image of truth in how you want to see yourself, and the kind of person you want to be. Seeing the ways others behave are helpful in deciding who YOU want to be, particularly in seeing others that have had trauma and/or difficulty and struggle in life and the positive ways you've seen THEM handle it. It is also useful to see the ways you think you AREN'T. Add any useful character traits that you would like to focus on in yourself, and add them to your Personal Avatar.

For example: Someone might observe someone they think is a great mom because you see them as patient, calm and fun. Keep in mind, you have an image of THEM, and likely they don't see themselves as wonderful as you do! They have their shortcomings as well. But it is useful to see the "mirrors" that are helping you see the person you want to be. Part of someone's image might now be to include, 'I see myself as a fun and patient mother, not in a hurry.' Add this to your personal avatar image and as you keep this image in the forefront of your mind (and even on paper so you can have it in front of you at all times), act based on this image during the day. What choices will you make that a fun patient mother would make?? How would a "fun patient mother" respond?

Why Play is important

Now that we've re-developed the idea of the self, let's start making use of that to have fun in life. Life is meant to be an experience, with some being more enjoyable than others. Play is what teaches young children through trial and experimentation and they enjoy the process. Why does that stop into adulthood? It's not because we wanted to, but because perceived expectations and encouragement for drive and ambition did. Ambition in itself is not a bad thing; it's because we've created our ambition according to cultural standards, rather than ambitions that come from a place of purpose within. Here's an idea. How about you stop doing what contributes to your unhappiness and follow your bliss? If you don't like what you're currently doing, make effort to try new things! MORE PLAY! Bring play into the balance of your life. Yes, I say that quite loudly because typically those of us with nagging anxiety, and using it incorrectly tend to over think, over analyze, and don't play enough. Living with this bigger, better, more mentality, we strive for more and soon our wants become needs. We become overwhelmed and exhausted, and largely it's because of our own making! We need to learn a little thing called faith, have some trust in the process, play and have fun. Everything happens for a reason and if we can remember that our lives are created based on our thoughts and the energy we put on things, it will be easier to remember that we want to cultivate our thoughts towards what we WANT, not what we don't want.

Claiming the Naming

Anxiety is not permanent unless you claim the name. When you start saying, "my anxiety..." like, "Oh, my anxiety is getting so bad. I can't handle it because I have anxiety", you are telling yourself and everyone around that you are not in control. When you hold onto it by possessing it, it's like negative prayer because you've claimed it as yours and you want to keep it that way. There is a big difference between acknowledging what IS, and where you intend to GO. "I'm getting better and better every day" is a great mantra to help rise above this hang up, as well as dropping off the words "my anxiety" or "I have anxiety". Voicing, if you have to at all, "I am healing from feelings of anxiety" is a better directive for your psyche, as well as the truth.

Claiming the Naming Exercise

Keep a pad of paper and small pen with you throughout the day.

Set your alarm clock to ring every hour.

Each time the alarm rings, write down what you were just thinking.

At the end of the day, look through your notes and identify where your words and thoughts have worked against you rather than for you.

Healing Anxiety symptoms and feelings takes WORK. And NO

one can do it for you but YOU. It's not just going to "go away".

Satisfaction's Healing Properties

We are always told gratitude is a key to having a good life, and it is. But I feel even more important, is learning the feeling of satisfaction. Satisfaction is like confident, content, gratitude. That through any and all things, you are ok. To learn satisfaction is to feel not only like you have no need in the present moment but that you are perfectly happy with that.

You may think you don't feel satisfaction now, but perhaps it is because you haven't been paying attention to it. You haven't been LOOKING for it. We have an incredible potential whenever we are faced with something that scares us, particularly about our health, to work for or against ourselves. When something is "wrong", we take notes, we google it, we see multiple practitioners for it, all looking for what's wrong.

Either way, whether there is right or wrong happening, you still have to live through it. It is my thought that it is a better use of time to enjoy being satisfied with all that we CAN be satisfied for than to live in misery. And certainly, gives our body more healing possibilities.

The Difference Between "Gratitude" and "Satisfaction"

They say when you are in struggle, or when you want to feel more joy in your life, or have had a tough road and you need to keep moving forward, to think of GRATITUDE. To live in the moment, paying attention to each and every thing you have to be grateful for. One idea is to create a gratitude journal or use a gratitude app, so that you can record the things you have to be thankful for. This way you can look back on this anytime you want, and it forces you to pay attention and shift the law of attraction to what you're wanting to see more of: the things you are grateful for.

Noticing gratitude, being aware of all of the things in your life you have to be thankful for is a wonderful new habit to be trained into. It is an excellent place to start: to pause and notice everything around you. But what if you don't truly feel it?

Let me explain what I discovered during my gratitude awareness intention and how it's changing me for the now.

I had heard gratitude was the way to ease out of depression, anxiety, and regain balance in a sense of living in the present. It is, and it does help. But when you're in a truly dark place of feeling like life is hard, you have struggles, and you have hurts and forgivenesses yet to heal and be had, "gratitude" can have an opposite effect. When I was in this very dark place, it did help to focus on the things I was grateful for, because I knew there were a lot of them. Here's the problem: I didn't FEEL grateful. I WAS grateful. I KNEW there were things I was grateful for. But what was also real was that I was SAD. And HURT. And ANGRY. And didn't know what to do. There was much I had to learn how to deal with in my new life and find happiness again, or ALLOW myself to be happy. Being aware of my gratefulness was a great first step. I have lists of all the things I was grateful for that surprised me when I thought that perhaps I truly didn't enjoy ANYTHING anymore. But when I didn't FEEL grateful, and knew I was feeling all of these other un-dealt with emotions, all this did was make me feel GUILTY that I couldn't be more happy. Noticing everything I should be grateful for, and all the good in my life, but it not changing how I FELT just made me feel like an awful person. What was so wrong with me that I couldn't feel that gratitude in the long-lasting way that brought happiness around again? It can be a hopeless place to be.

Not to mention what if you really DON'T feel grateful? When I was in the wheelchair, for example, or once our infant Solomon was born early and sleeping, I didn't WANT to see the silver lining. Even though people would say "yes, but you still have other healthy children", or "at least you're still alive". It was almost a pandering condescension rather than the well-meaning sentiments I knew they intended. But there is something about acknowledging the fact that you just, maybe, in that moment, DON'T feel grateful.

Enter "satisfaction":

Satisfaction is the FEELING of the gratitude. It is the contented peace and ENJOYMENT that comes from acknowledging the things you are grateful for. Training yourself to notice your gratitude is a NOTICING and and AWARENESS and sets the stage for one to see anew, rather than see the things that were causing discontent previously. But NOTICING is different from FEELING.

Even if you train yourself to recognize how gratitude FEELS, it still does not translate into what it means in your life. Take it a step further: once you can FEEL gratitude, it means what in your life? Feeling grateful gives you Satisfaction and isn't that what you were searching for? When you think of it, why are you reaching towards ANY good feeling emotion? If you follow the white rabbit, is it because you are looking for peace? happiness? joy? contentedness? For me, the FEELING of satisfaction is all of these. It is a peace and gratitude, a quiet contentedness of the ENJOYMENT of how all of these gratitudes I notice FEEL in my life.

Here is my suggestion: be open to feeling your satisfactions. To not only acknowledge and notice ALL that is in your life "good" and "bad", but that when you DO feel gratitude and thankfulness, to notice how it feels in the body; to notice the contentedness, the peace, and the enjoyment.... which is all what I believe you might actually be searching for in the first place.

If you don't feel gratitude, it can sometimes be almost a guilty punishing you can feel towards yourself. When you don't feel "satisfied", it's not a statement about YOU, in fact, it's an opportunity to give you ACTION. What can you do to increase satisfaction?

Then you can set goals. Not goals like you've heard to do like new year's resolutions. When your life feels dull, confusing, boring, stressful, and even challenging, you can give yourself a goal, which is going to make you feel like you are moving forward SOMEHOW.

Happy Action Exercise

Find something you enjoy, that does bring satisfaction, and vow to do more of it. For example, if you like to read, develop a reading challenge for yourself to read a number of books in a given time frame.

If sewing brings you satisfaction, create a challenge to sew every day for a half an hour. Or sew a new pattern each month. Or buy 12 new patterns at the store, challenging yourself to do at least one of each before the year is up.

Create a countdown chain, a crossoff chart, or a list, so that when you finish it, you can acknowledge the satisfaction you feel in completion and celebrate it through seeing it tangibly. Take time to FEEL how "satisfied" feels.

Even if you are a stay at home mom feeling bored with monotony, or the challenges in raising kids, you can always come up with a way to move yourself forward. For example: if you feel like you haven't had time to get through cleaning and organizing your house. Come up with a challenge to complete it.

It will give you focus and something to pay attention to, which will make you have a plan for your day. Draw a map of your house. Take a day for each room. The challenge is to clean and organize each room on the day that you marked it. Then color it in on your map. You will have something to look forward to when you wake up each morning by knowing what your day is about, and the feeling of satisfaction once it's completed.

Feeling a lack of 'satisfaction' just means that you haven't had a plan for your own happiness and have not created a life in which your satisfaction is paramount.

Feeling 'satisfaction' means you have an acknowledgement of the gratitude you feel through the sense of peace and contentedness you feel. When it comes down to it, it's not about our circumstances, our situations, or what we own. It's about how we FEEL, and I think we all want to feel happy and joyful. Satisfaction is the feeling you have while enjoying the things you have created in your life. Feeling 'satisfaction' is the manifestation that happens when you have decided to value your happiness and have made a plan to spend your time in it.

Gratitude Journal Exercise

Keep a daily journal in which you look back over the day and write down all the things, big and small, that you feel gratitude for.

Don't write a journal like a diary, detailing your whole day, but as a bullet list, so you can quickly and easily see all the good things to focus on.

Look at these pages when you are having a low time to help you pull out of the slump.

But also sit back after writing each day, and allow yourself to feel a deep satisfaction with being grateful for your life and the feeling that "all is well". Even if just for a moment, gradually those moments add up. When you are training yourself to look for these feelings during the day, you will pay attention to them. While we have used this method used previously and elsewhere, I want to take it a step further. When you are starting to notice throughout the day these moments of gratitude, we tend to move through it so fast. Instead, stop. Take notice. Look at whatever attracted your attention and joy. Feel how the feeling feels in your body and where. When you do this, you will begin to recognize the feeling of satisfaction and allow more of these moments throughout your day. You will be literally experiencing the joys of life throughout the day, realizing they are most often not in the large events like new purchases, jobs, or possessions. All experiences are fleeting, big ones and little. They don't last. They only last in our memory of feeling, so when you're in one, be sure to use all five senses to secure it into your memory.

Let me give you an example. I was holding the hand of my five-year-old and he was so excited from the experience he had and he looked up at me so in love and joyfully, and in this moment, I was smart enough to know not to rush through it. Suddenly getting him to the car wasn't what mattered anymore. Instead, I really looked at his smile, his face and his eyes, I smiled back, felt the warmth of his little hand, and felt the satisfaction of seeing my happy little guy in my heart. I knelt down and took in his excited hug and took the time to share in his joy. That memory is more secure in my mind now than if I had simply said a passing word and continued hurrying him to the car. In that moment, I was truly living. THIS is living, folks.

8 Anxiety is a Disease of Separation

Anxiety is a dis-ease of separation. It is commonly believed that anxiety is an entirely personal thing that must be healed by diving into one's own mind and the imbalanced chemistry that resides there. I do not however believe this, however, you don't have to believe my opinions, it's biology. It is well understood that a sense of belonging is a very basic human need. This may not be logical in the grand scheme of bodily needs, but a healthy psyche is essential to physical needs. This sense of belonging doesn't even have to come from people, but could be a sense of belonging to a cause, animals, an organization, a routine. It is a feeling that comes from being around and accepted into a flow of like minded-ness, where you are able to be in harmony with your core values. I believe the trappings of anxiety come from a place of being so far removed from the feeling of connection with anything in the world around them, including themselves. The gap between this experience and wanting to feel at peace with connection to SOMETHING and a place of belonging is where anxiety lives. Individuals will try to fill this void with action, something that will make them feel busy and worthwhile and notable. As we've seen, this results in the anxiety of overwhelm and overburden we've been discussing so far, yet without the fulfilled feeling one is searching for. People will go to great lengths to search for this feeling of connection, which is why I say there is danger in anxiety being a contagious dis-ease. Out of this innate sense of belonging and wholeness by being part of a group who are like us and share our situations, there is the risk that the group becomes a group of people that bond together IN ILLNESS, rather than IN WHOLENESS. Others may hide from this sense of belongingness when they feel anxiety because they feel as if they just DON'T belong, staying singularly in illness. People can "belong' in alone-ness, but when it's because they are hiding, it's anxiety driven and NOT the path out. Our innate need of belonging is really our soul's ability to "auto-correct", able to turn on the dashboard light that tells us we are off track. This innate ability makes us also really good at spotting things that don't belong - which is why you feel the anxiety you feel - something doesn't belong. See how your body is just trying to help you? You can prolong the pain, or learn to adapt. Since the limbic system in the brain is what is responsible for our feelings, but not our ability to communicate how we are feeling, is why it's hard to put "anxiety" feelings into words, but is also the system responsible for how we know something is right; it's because "it just feels right", the guidance system we should be following. When people are making decisions with their rational brain, inevitably this is where "overthinking" comes in to play. If we want to guide ourselves from that which is raw and real to us, then we need to employ the "feels right" guidance system rather than all all the attention that is placed on "thinking" it out. Because we've been taught to THINK and PLAN we often don't trust our ability to feel out if something is right or not and so we rely on outside sources, indicators, and persuasions, all of which can take us away from our true selves, expanding that gap where anxiety thrives.

While the self must be understood in silence and individually grown, healing comes ultimately from a place of feeling connected - to a group, to individuals, to silence, to nature, to a cause, to a purpose. When one returns to a state of balance and feeling of wholeness, they can hear this inner calling more clearly and can then enjoy the satisfaction of being in flow and is less prone to feeling the sways of anxiety. Some feel connected being part of a group, some feel connected in the stillness of themselves, but the truth remains: one must have an approval of one's own self.

Acts of Service

The feeling of anxiety makes our four walls feel very small. I've said it many times that I think we are too often in our own little box of comfort and that one of the best things we could do for ourselves and others would be to experience other cultures, to find who we are amongst the world and how can we do that if we've only seen our small box? We see only with the limited eyes of where we have lived and had our being. Seeing parts of the world that differ from where we currently reside has the power to challenge our concepts that the way "we" do things is the only right way. This releases feelings of anxiety because there is acceptance for "different", and the understanding that there is not one right way to be.

I fully believe that when you are feeling down, sorry for yourself, or off track, go find someone else that you can help. Of course, you are allowed to feel how you are feeling and there is benefit to staying there for a time, until you learn the lesson you were intended to learn. Staying there longer is a victimized mentality, keeping you dis-eased, and depriving yourself and the world of your Greatness Within. Engaging in our own states once again keeps us in our comfort box and the view from above is each of us cramped in our own tiny little boxes of our own making.

"Self-absorption in all its forms kills empathy, let alone compassion. When we focus on ourselves, our world contracts as our problems and preoccupations loom large. But when we focus on others, our world expands", Daniel Goleman, author of "Social Intelligence".

Understanding life from another's point of view allows us to re-shift our focus of comparison. I said earlier that anxiety is a dis-ease of separation, healed by community. Once we can put ourselves in others' shoes and live to accept each person as they are with no judgement, we re-instate a sense of compassion, which is one of the reasons we have become so sheltered and over-burdened in the first place. Collectively we've forgotten about compassion, about connection, and eventually we end up in seclusion rather than that feeling of being at one with life. This, I believe, is the greatest reason we feel this sense of dis-connect, struggle, and overwhelm. Instead of feeling the connection of all that is and seeing how we are a part of it, we are judging and comparing ourselves on or mobile phones and social media accounts, at work, at school and the PTA, and then endlessly trying to make ourselves beat out, have more and do more than the next person. The problem is, that never brings the satisfaction and contentment we're looking for and so we have to keep it up: both the image we've created and doing even more, bringing about the very overwhelm and anxiety we are trying to then spend tons of money on medications and counseling sessions to overcome. With all of this striving for more, we forget the very core of who we are, which is why I make the suggestion to develop your Personal Avatar: to get back to a place of being with yourself, with what matters, your core values and the kind of person you want to BE, not so much what you want to ACHIEVE.

We can expand outside of our comfort box by visiting and experiencing other places, and we can expand our comfort boxes by serving others. By seeing outside ourselves and our own needs we can challenge our beliefs about how victimized we really are. Besides the good this self-reflection does for us, we at the same time benefit others which has its own intrinsic value. In addition, serving others feels good, and has the power to rewire the same connections that cause imbalanced chemistry, this time swaying in our favor.

The Comfort Box

If we can't go to that extent, then at least to discover other social situations or engage in new experiences. This can be done alone as well as in a social group until you have healed the traumas and/or self-worth issues that lead to social anxiety. This does not need to stop you from trying new things, which can be done right in your own home or community, until you are ready. Taking baby steps is fine as long as you are truly moving forward; jumping right into Your Personal Avatar, the person you want to be and just beginning, is another way. Either way, we can learn lesson from Jim Carrey's movie, "Yes Man" in which he must say yes to everything. While of course that is an exaggeration, the idea is that life happens when you are open, flexible, and adaptable, without interfering with flow by trying to control everything out of fear. Remember, you could be keeping things away that are meant for your personal growth and keeping yourself away from what could be enjoyable experiences. The world is a playground of experience within which, our souls find themselves, through experiences good and bad. Even having "negative" experiences expand us as people and give us the opportunity to practice who we want to be. It is not logic and reason but dreams and aspirations that get us to try new things so if you are having a hard time making decisions it is again because you are analyzing and overthinking, rather than feeling and moving in a positive direction for yourself. If we always thought rationally and logically, we would not have small business, or new engineering, or even chemistry and biology experiments to cure disease -because nobody would expand out of the comfort box.

I mentioned the comfort box in previous chapters as one of the most dangerous places in which you can live. Most often the struggle of overwhelm, burden, stress, and resulting anxiety with all of the responsibilities and expectations we are trying to meet, that understandably, our schedules get jam-packed. This is why it is essential to first understand WHO you are and what you are trying to do, the person you are becoming with the Personal Avatar exercise (all exercises mentioned are available at drfoodie.live or in this book), and then sort out what your responsibilities truly are with the Responsibility Exercise and the three Expectation Exercises.

With a schedule that is too packed, we don't leave room for zen, for stillness, for flexibility, and we become controlling over our environments and the people in them so that MORE doesn't happen. Which, interestingly enough pushes away MORE of the good stuff too! This sense of needing to control starts a slippery slope involving our relationships with our children, our spouse, and friendships. We don't allow for change because we have developed what feels "comfortable" to us. We have built the walls of our "comfort box" up around ourselves, making it very hard for others to come in and help, and even harder for you to see beyond the walls to see your way out.

We must step outside of our comfort box. Feel the flow of the day rather than the restrictions and limitations our current "to do" schedule has necessitated. Stepping out of your comfort box allows new experiences, things you haven't tried before and engages the free creator we truly are. It allows things we HAVEN'T planned for to pop up to show us who we really are.

Even if you feel like you can't change your schedule right now, you can:

1. Tidy up your expectations and responsibilities, with the Expectations and Responsibility Exercises

2. Get busy volunteering. Find a way you can relieve someone else's true needs. I know, it feels like we already do this all the time for our families. That's not the same

thing. Often times you're tending to their WANTS, which is very different than serving a soup kitchen to people who don't have any food.

3. You CAN try new experiences. Sitting in our comfort box for too long has our minds thinking OUT on an experience from our limited point of view. Our THOUGHTS make an assumption on the value and worth of a new experience before we even try it. Our logical minds are ever in high gear telling us what makes "sense" or not, before we've even gotten to just have the experience. And soon we're talking ourselves out of everything. Get out of your comfort box; if you had nothing to fear, what kinds of things would you do? Use the prompt on the following page for help with this. Let your list be long and exhaustive, and don't let your mind do any filtering; just write it down!

Amanda Plevell

The No Fear Exercise:

Mark Twain was right. "The fear of death follows from the fear of life.

A man who lives his life fully is prepared to die at any time."

Those in anxiety work to fight it.

For this exercise use this prompt to brainstorm and list EVERYTHING you can think of.: "If nothing scared me, I would…."

_____

_____

_____

_____

_____

_____

_____

_____

_____

_____

Unbound

Congratulations! You just wrote your REAL bucket list. These are the things to aspire to, rather than an "I Wish" list, which is what many bucket lists become. Being the person, you want to be is the best bucket list you can have. These now are the things that you get out your daily and yearly calendar and plan into your life, otherwise life just passes you by while you forget to live. The next step is to plan each of these into your calendar. We've put together, along with instructions for their use, a yearly calendar and our Am/Pm Planner designed just for this purpose...to help you really achieve what you are looking for out of life, and to reduce the responsibilities you've accumulated to purposeful ones for your life missions.

Curing Anxiety

When we talk about anxiety, and how to "cure" anxiety or "get rid of it", essentially you never will from that mindset because it is not something to "get rid of". It is a warning signal, a sign, a directional cue to make some changes. This is why anxiety is not an epidemic, it's our greatest opportunity for change! Look how great the world would be if everyone accessed their Greatness Within and lived from a place of loving decisions rather than fear decisions.

Because we're not there yet, sure, I have a list of supplements and techniques that can help, but my list doesn't include the typical "tried and true" strategies we've all read on the pinterest boards, you know the ones: Breathe, Vitamin B, Vitamin D, Magnesium, Get a massage, Learn to relax, manage your stress.......All well and good ideas, but about what really gets to the core of what our beings need?

The list I rely on the most is one that reminds us of our connections. My list puts us in a humble place within the world of being observant to life around us. With our hustle bustle competing lives, we THINK we are seeing life around us by

DOING life and watching what everyone else is doing, but we forget that we are watching life on a manmade stage, with manmade structures, wearing man made clothes, using man made ideals and illusions about success and necessity. And we've done all this with no consideration for the destruction of life. I will tell you what. That's not life. Do you feel like you're living? All this illusion has made us forget who we are, and our sense of worth gets questioned by ourselves, meaning we have to strive for still more. We forget the simplicity of life, like what life was like when we were kids, where play and discovery was our only concern, and a hike or a bike ride was our greatest ambition and we explored the magic of what an egg could do in your mud pie. Only now, today's kids don't even know what that feels like as we've already started them on our anxiety/overwhelm path of expectation and burden at younger and younger ages.

    Connecting with real life reminds us of the simplicity of living, which has the power to wipe away feelings of anxiety and overwhelm in an instant. All it takes is dropping the act and remembering life. Here's my list, but really, all lists aside, the point is to engage and pay attention. To observe. To listen and see without judgement. To clear the mind and just notice what we can learn from watching nature, the only being that does not bow to our man made "rules". Certainly, you can use these in a moment of situational anxiety or panic attack, but keep in mind, I'm talking about using these techniques daily, regularly, and as a lifestyle to release the burden of anxiety altogether. I'm not talking about just using these techniques situationally, but continuously and repeatedly.

Amanda Plevell

My Anxiety Cures List

- Look at the clouds. Notice them and watch them move

- Take a looking walk. What do you see? Don't just walk unobservantly. Pay attention to textures, sounds, feelings. Try to engage all 5 senses as you walk and notice the life around you. Do you see how that plant still grew through the concrete crack? Do you see how the tree struck with lightning bent but started growing in a new direction?

- Watch the water. See how it moves, and what moves with it.

- Watch the wind in the trees.

- Watch nature. Every bit and piece of it.

- Get down low. Just like how when we drive on the interstate, we are "passersby", missing all the life going on in the cities we pass through. If we get own low and watch in the grass, we see life at its very smallest; things we would normally miss in our hurry to just get somewhere.

- Pay attention to something you've never paid attention to before. Watch people and how they are handling their moments, without word or judgement. Watch your child play. Really watch them, their facial expressions, the way they figure things out.

- Look at something with a magnifying glass. Have you ever seen the veins on a leaf? Or turned up a cornstalk and noticed how the roots are all pre-arranged in a whorl pattern? How did that happen if we DIDN'T live in a cosmically, divinely organized world? There is a plan, an organization too great it couldn't be by coincidence. There was a plan that made that whorl pattern so that it could be it's strongest in wind and weather. Look at the intricacies of tropical flowers. How could that work of art be at random? You are not at random, either.

- Find someone you can help. Not because they are less than, but because you can. They're really helping you, anyway.

- Do something you used to do as a kid. Play, run, blow bubbles, make a mudpie.

- Watch it snow, rain, blow. Just pull up a chair and a cup of cocoa with no sense of time frame. Get mesmerized in undiscovered action.

- Make footprints. In the mud, in the snow, in the sand.

- Feel the sun on your skin and take notice.

- Laugh. Really laugh. Pay attention to how your body feels.

- Read.

- Draw.

- Look at art created by others and see it. What was the artist thinking? Why did they use the flow, texture, and colors that they did? Can you feel what they were feeling? Connect.

- Listen to music. Dance. Move your body.

- Be an anomaly to what everyone thinks you "should" be.

- Start exclaiming over the amazing good in people, instead of celebrities and social media accounts.

- Stop watching other people's lives and start living your

own.

- Say yes to new experiences, step out of the box of comfort and trust yourself to learn courage. To wake everyday with the idea that no matter WHAT happens, to face it with determination, joy and bravery.

- Find out what makes you happy and do more of those things. Use my calendar and AM/PM Journal to plan for these.

- Keep a gratitude journal. Not just to write down 5 things you're grateful for, but because the feeling of gratitude will become a place that you live more often, the more time you spend there.

Zen Techniques

We plan too much into our day and forget to go with the flow of life. This makes us in-flexible, rigid, and always running to be "on-time". This is why we do the calendar exercise (the one I mentioned on our Unbound website VIP section) to plan out first what really matters to us, to keep ourselves whole so that we are acting with a whole self at all times. Practicing the zen technique of mindfulness is important because it trains your mind to do one thing at a time. In a state of anxiety or overwhelm we find ourselves continuously multi-tasking, rushing and scurrying. This confuses the mind, making it hard to stop the mind from running wherever it wants whenever it wants. This type of training is hard to stop. The fact that we CAN multi-task is an amazing ability of the mind in case of situations where we have to think fast and adapt. But the lifesaving times we would need to do this have greatly diminished over evolution and we are using this tool as a daily occurrence, rather than the fail-safe it was meant to be. Zen techniques remind your mind to live focused.

These zen techniques will remind you to be in a mindset of space and time and peace as you are moving through your day.

Zen Techniques

1. Do one thing at a time
2. Do it slowly and deliberately
3. Do it completely
4. Do less
5. Put space between things
6. Develop rituals
7. Designate time for certain things

8. Devote time to sitting

9. Smile and serve others

10. Think about what is necessary

11. Live simply

12. Be grateful

13. Notice feelings of satisfaction

***

Ultimately, we are all here for a purpose, on purpose. We are here to discover ourselves, and how that self may be of benefit to others by making a unique imprint on the world around us. We tend to make life too complicated and end up creating the very struggle we are trying to avoid. Trying to live a life we believe we "should" want to live ends up in the hustle scurrying breathless life of overwhelm, stress, and burden. Living in this continuous pace of learned anxiety removes us from the experiences of satisfaction ripe and ready for us to experience. When we know ourselves well, understand what makes us "us", our core values and the kind of people we want to be, it's easier to make choices for ourselves. This puts us at a better, stronger, more confident place to be able to play well the other roles we have chosen for ourselves. When we come from a place of within, the universe works in our favor. Trying from a place you are NOT brings struggle and frustration. So when things go wrong, learning from your feelings, including those of anxiety are ultimately a way to identify more with who you really are, and who you really want to be.

There is only one life that you get to live and the time here is fleeting. When you release yourself from the things you DON'T want in your life, you make room on your bucket list for the things you DO. Life is meant for living and being happy. What are you waiting for? Even the tasks of the day to day can be satisfying if you are coming from a good strong sense of self and determine that all life is good. It's time to make your life one that is RIPE with experiences of your own making. You can choose to take your hard lessons as a reason NOT to rise, forever remaining a victim, or you can use these lessons to learn from, truly becoming.....Unbound.

About the Author

Amanda Plevell, PhD, CNHP is just like you. Living with her five guys and four pets with a home to manage, homeschool, and a community clinic she knows well the burden of overwhelm and anxiety. It was only after immense struggle herself and witnessing it happening in clients and friends that she decided on a new call to action, changing life for herself and others in the process. Having worked with a client list in the thousands over the past 14 years, she is a master at converting the impossible and creating life from chaos, helping people all over the globe rethink overwhelm and burden to get back to themselves and a life they love living. A Natural Health Practitioner, Wellness Advocate and Educator, Author, Speaker, and Trainer, a most popularly followed Intuitive Business Trainer and Program Developer, she usually says yes as long as it fits her image and doesn't distort her balance. She is a recognized authority on Concept Pathology, the psychology of nourishment, and their effects on healing. Author of over 28 natural health and self development books, Amanda is well sought after in the arenas of education, wellness and health, and business development. Her bestselling books include such titles as " The Success Conditioning Work it Out Book", "The Genesis Code", "I Am Success", "The Energy of Divorce", and "Clean Your Plate". You can find her on Facebook and on Instagram.com/apdrfoodie.

Now you can experience UnBound at an even more personal level with our Customized Success Kit. It's Easy! Take our quick quiz, and it will generate a personalized kit with activities and exercises that are the most beneficial for you. Go to www.buildyourownbucketlist.com to begin.

Don't forget to join our Live Coaching! And get real life help walking through the steps to kick anxiety from YOUR bucket list!

Unbound

UnBound: Raw and Real Plans to Kick Anxiety From Your Bucket List.

My mission in life is to help people find their Greatness Within. My desire in EVERYTHING I DO is to raise mass consciousness, by being the best I can be and encouraging people to do the same, it's the only way we will all be better! One of the ways I do this is as a PhD'd Natural Health Practitioner and in my clinic I work with people with physical symptoms and manifestations, but always, always is the physical problem in relation to some other struggle internally. "Anxiety" is such a pervasive problem right now and we need to take a break in regular health programming to truly help people with it, but here's the real problem: we made the feelings of anxiety into a THING, as if it's a BAD part of us, when really feelings and expression of anxiety are the body's natural and normal response as a tool and defense mechanism. The VERY REAL problem is the number of people that feel feelings of anxiety, are really feeling overwhelm, overburdened and discontent, BECAUSE THEY KNOW THE LIVES THEY ARE LIVING in comparison to THE LIVES THEY ARE MEANT TO are vastly different, and the gap between is the "anxiety" they are feeling. I believe people innately know they have a greater soul purpose, but the societal pressure to be somebody takes us away from this, compounding the layers of untruths on top of us, creating the burden we feel. I feel it is absolutely imperative people understand that this anxietyis a call to be your greatness, to live a life that manifests your soul potential, and in this way completes the mission of why I do anything - to raise mass consciousness. I have self-published many books, as workbooks to help people improve, but I want this book to reach people, to truly make an impact and cause the ripples that create change!

12 Week Unbound Course

NOW! UnBound comes to you in a series of 12 Lessons

Straight to Your Inbox!

Get further insights and personalized self-led and directed learning through all of the

RAW AND REAL PLANS TO KICK ANXIETY FROM YOUR BUCKET LIST

Search "UnBound 12 Week" on www.drfoodie.live to begin!

Made in the USA
Middletown, DE
09 March 2019